Your Amazing Itty Bitty™ Fitness for Healing Pain Book

15 Steps to a New Way to Exercise for Pain Relief and Physical Repair

Meg Margolis

Published by Itty Bitty™ Publishing
A subsidiary of S & P Productions, Inc.

Printed in the United States of America

Itty Bitty Publishing
311 Main Street, Suite D
El Segundo, CA 90245
(310) 640-8885

ISBN: 978-1-959964-76-6

Finally, Pain Relief From Within!

Discover the Power of Healing Movement

Are you in Excruciating pain? You don't have to suffer!

Even the most painful areas in your body can move freely without strain when you exercise from a position of comfort and support. Your body is designed to heal itself, and with the right techniques, you can reach total relief and speed up that process.

In this transformative Itty Bitty™ book, Meg Margolis will teach you how to:

- Relieve pain effectively and naturally
- Use placement breathing for comfort and healing
- Perform muscle movements that enhance flexibility, strength, and endurance
- And so much more!

If you're ready to take control of your pain and get lasting relief, this Itty Bitty™ book is your guide to a life of comfort and healing. Pick up a copy today!

"Dr. Arthur White, orthopedic surgeon for Joe Montana, endorses Margolis' exercise program. In some cases, he says proper exercise can eliminate the need for surgery."

~ *San Francisco Chronicle*

Praise for A New Way To Exercise Program

"Meg Margolis assisted my wife's recovery from severe back disease, unsuccessful back surgery, and prolonged bed rest. She is a very talented and inventive teacher of the difficult and complex exercises required for the re-education of muscles and the alteration of body balance and mechanics, which contribute to recovery from back disease."

~ Dr. Alan C. Aisenberg, Harvard Medical School, Associate Professor of Medicine

"Fitness For Living is more likely to benefit than most physical therapy programs."

~ Dr. William Clark, Medical Director, CA Workers' Compensation Appeals Board

"Since Meg has been working with my women's basketball program, the results have been stunning and immediate. My team has more quickness and agility, which has led them to run faster and jump higher."

~ Michel Fulton, Head Coach Women's Basketball Team, College of Marin

"I had done it all, and nothing was working. Doctors, out of despair, referred me to Meg. I started getting better immediately… It didn't take long to redevelop muscles in a way that was totally foreign to me; no weights, no strain, no 'no pain, no gain'."

~ Roger Stillwell, Chicago Bears, All-Pro American Football Player

Dedication

This book is dedicated to you, the reader. It will teach you how to have control and power over your own physical pain.

I love sharing this information with the world. I am especially grateful to Maggie Lettvin, my teacher at MIT, who encouraged me to see beyond the work she was already teaching. Maggie sent Ruth Corwin, PhD, all the way to California from Cambridge, Massachusetts, to work with me. And to Kaiser Permanente for sending me coach Tony Blandino, who comes from a long line of Blandino doctors, pro ball players, pharmacists, and teachers.

Ruth and Tony have been both my students and co-teachers since 1984, giving me the necessary support and encouragement to present this information to you.

Stop by our Itty Bitty™ website to find interesting information regarding DIY pain relief and physical repair.

www.IttyBittyPublishing.com

Or visit Meg Margolis at:

https://painreliefexercise.com

Table of Contents

Step 15. Standing and Jiggling for Circulation, Leg Cramps, and Tension Release

Introduction

The good news is that even the most painful areas in your body can easily move without straining or pain when you exercise from a fully supported position of comfort.

This book will teach you how to position yourself for pain relief and physical repair, along with the exercises that use your breathing muscle movements for building new flexibility, strength, and endurance.

If your injured tissue is allowed to expand, contract, and relax without having to strain for the motion and if the movement is easy enough to be repeated without pain or irritation, then you are in control of your physical exercise program for pain relief and physical repair.

Finding a new way to exercise encourages physical repair responses to interrupt and change progressive body breakdown. Your body works to repair itself every moment. Even after death, the body continues to change, only slower.

You will learn within these pages how to exercise the extraordinary physical repair and pain relief capacity you were born with. Correct information reverses the hopelessness of believing you have to live in pain.

Step 1
Support What Hurts to Stop Your Pain

Pain changes when strategically placed supports are utilized under all the different parts of your body. By transferring the body weight of injured areas to the specific supports, your body relaxes stressed and/or strained muscles.

1. A fully supported pelvic tilt relaxes hip flexors, renews joint spacing, and lengthens the muscles at your lower back to relieve your pain.
2. Using properly positioned supports releases your leg muscles, pelvis, and spine, so that nerve roots can heal.
3. When you support your head and arms, weight is lifted from your neck, shoulders, and upper back.

When you lie on your back supported from head to toe, your spine decompresses, and your body releases pain. Positioning this way allows you to exercise for repair and release without irritating existing problems. This allows you to comfortably build endurance, strength, and flexibility.

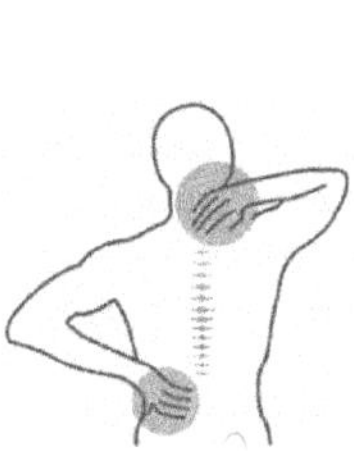

More About Stopping Pain by Supporting What Hurts

- Releasing the pressure of your body weight in gravity lightens the workload on muscle fibers and joint spaces.
- Belly weight drops into the cradle of the pelvis, no longer creating strain on the lumbar spine. This lessens your pot belly.
- Digestive problems, cramps, intestinal issues, and muscle spasms will receive greater circulation and space for better functionality, because blood is carried more effectively throughout your circulatory system, which delivers oxygen to every area, thus releasing muscle spasms and feeding every cell and physical function.

Step 2
Change the Message From Pain to Comfort

Position yourself for healing comfort to improve pain-free range of motion. Fully supported muscles can move in ways that unsupported muscles cannot.

1. Fully supported muscles will relax and move the distance they were designed to go.
2. Pain-free range of supported motion activates physical rest and repair.
3. Supported positioning gives even long-term painful muscles the ability to fully expand, contract, and relax without strain or pain.

Exercise is ineffective when it does not include the soft and spacious motions of rest, repair, and relaxation. Physical rest is uninterrupted movement.

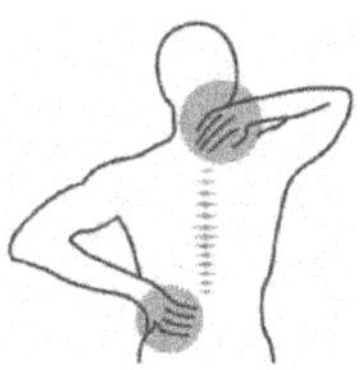

More About Changing the Message from Pain to Comfort

- Fully supported exercise changes the chemistry of pain by increasing your range of pain-free movement.
- Pain-free movement naturally increases as a result of fully supported exercise, which improves fluid circulation.
- Pain, inflammation, spasms, and anxiety change as blood and lymph circulation improve.
- Improved blood circulation expands oxygen delivery. Oxygen is carried in the bloodstream. Cells cannot repair or live without oxygen.
- Repeating the exercise floods your nervous system with messages of relief and repair while sending, receiving, and recording them as new habits.

Step 3
Where There's Pain There's Loss of Movement

Whether pain problems develop over time or happen in an instant, loss of movement is at the heart of pain. Pain is a response, not an inherent state. Something happens to make your body hurt.

1. Nerve compression and degenerating discs are results of muscle motions that have slowed down or stopped altogether.
2. Loss of muscle movement triggers a chain reaction that restricts joint movement, blood flow, lymph circulation, and the removal of waste products.
3. Motion is the language of your body. It carries, sends, and delivers all messages.

Movement is your key protector against pain. Every system—respiratory, circulatory, digestive, muscular, skeletal, immune, and nervous is a changing structure of individual parts that expand, contract, or relax.

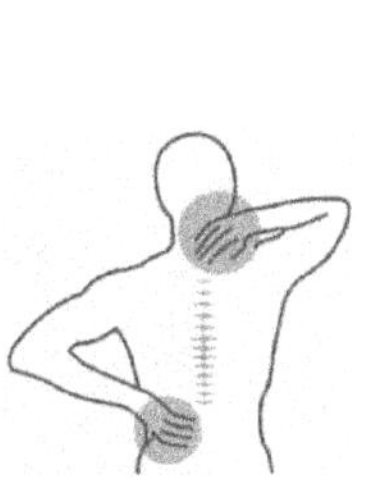

More About Where There's Pain There's Loss of Movement

Movement is a constant in the body. Healthy cells never stop moving unless there's a problem.

- The expanded range of supported motion during exercise produces and delivers healing messages to every function and structure of the body.
- When your body gets even a little bit of pain relief, it will continue to move in that direction.
- Muscles expand and lengthen for flexibility; they contract and shorten for strength, and soften to open for rest and relaxation.
- Painful muscles have a hard time resting. Pain problems are notifications that limited movement has settled in.

Step 4
Supported Muscles Break the Holding Power of Pain

If compressing pressure of body weight in gravity doesn't bear down on enclosed soft tissues and embedded blood and lymphatic vessels, muscles immediately recover their ability to relax and move without straining.

1. In your supported position of comfort, the weight of each body part acts as passive traction. Passive traction is where decompression makes space for soft tissue to expand, relax, and contract without pain.
2. Without stretch or strain, supported muscle fibers lengthen, and joint spaces bend and open.
3. Even after years of living in pain, supported movement can break the holding power of pain.

From a fully-supported exercise position, muscles expand to give bones, connecting tissue, joints, and fluids movement that interrupts the holding power of pain.

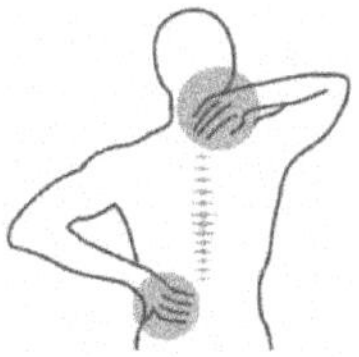

More About Supported Muscles: Break the Holding Power of Pain

Exercises using supported positions for lengthening muscles avoid overstretching or pulling injured and/or painful areas.

- The rebuilding key that facilitates healing change is exercise that doesn't cause pain or strain.
- Exercising inside your comfort zone can build physical ability right where the problem is to develop protective strength and flexibility without irritating existing injury sites.

Step 5
Breathing Muscle Movements

Breathing muscles are the only muscles that attach to and are responsible for moving vertebrae up and down your spine. Breathing muscles are also responsible for moving ribs, collarbone, sternum, chest, shoulders, shoulder blades, upper back, lower back, and pelvis.

1. Breathing muscles give your hips, belly, waist, and posture their shape and tone.
2. When breathing muscles move normally, they feed discs and protect against degenerative changes.
3. Movement of supported breathing muscles interrupts the wear and tear of arthritis, herniation, sciatica, and scoliosis.

Breathing muscle movements fuel relief and repair responses, relax spasms, maintain soft connecting tissues, bend joints, maintain and build bone density, deliver blood, and circulate lymph fluid to every cell in the body.

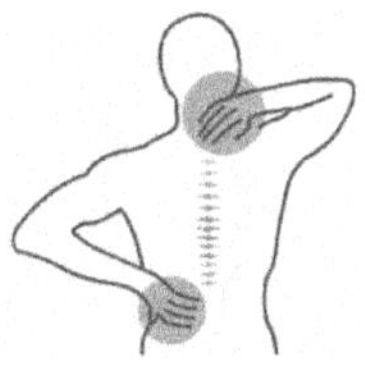

More About Breathing Muscle Movements

- The more you hurt, the more you need the breathing muscle movements you had at birth. Have you ever noticed how easily babies' backs and bottoms move when they breathe?
- Babies make full use of their breathing muscles to discharge stress and recover from excitement by utilizing crying, yawning, tears, sounds, and laughter responses.
- The long sigh after a good cry is your nervous system returning to balance. Yawning is a response to the need for a new supply of oxygen.
- The motion of laughter relaxes artery wall muscles, easing stress on the heart muscle as it pumps blood through 75,000 miles of circulatory routes.

Step 6
Immune Enhancement

Supported muscular breathing exercises give bones the necessary motions to produce blood marrow cells. White blood cells are the primary workers of your immune system. Red blood cells carry oxygen, which you can't live without.

1. As muscles contract on the exhale, they squeeze the walls of lymph-carrying vessels, supplying lymph fluid to every cell.
2. White blood cells detect and pick up heavy metals, bacteria, and viruses. Debris removal is the first step in recovering health.
3. After a long inhale, sigh, or yawn, the thoracic duct opens for lymph access to every cell.

Clusters of lymph nodes protect you by detoxing and filtering waste products to be carried off to eliminative organs. These nodes are deep inside your pelvis, at your underarms, along the sides of your neck, and up and down your spine and legs.

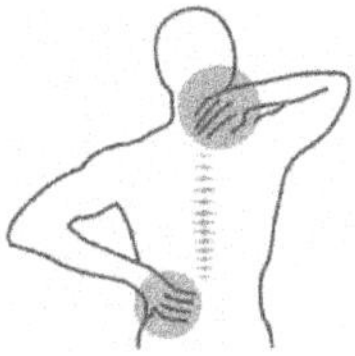

More About Immune Enhancement

- The expanding, contracting, and relaxing movements of supported exercise provide the stress-free physical motion necessary for immune rebuilding.
- Pain, inflammation, and anxiety improve when waste products from irritable states of mind and body are relieved from congestion in soft tissues and joint spaces.
- Flood painful damaged areas with reparative motions that move your body in the direction you want it to go.
- Fully-supported exercise relieves the compressing pressures of body weight in gravity and takes the workload off soft tissues and joint spaces. This encourages the physical repair responses you were born with, which interrupt progressive body breakdown.

Step 7
Shoes, Misinformation, and Society's Influence

Learned misinformation wears away at the inherent physical protections of muscles, joints, connecting tissues, circulatory movements, nervous system responses, and immune functions.

1. Overcoming the effects of misbelief is more complicated than learning how to correctly care for your body.
2. The repair response to repeated full, strain-free movement is mistakenly called miraculous or unusual instead of the ordinary, correct expectation.
3. The truth is that blood vessels regrow, fluids circulate, nerves make new connections, and supported exercise relieves pain and repairs muscles.

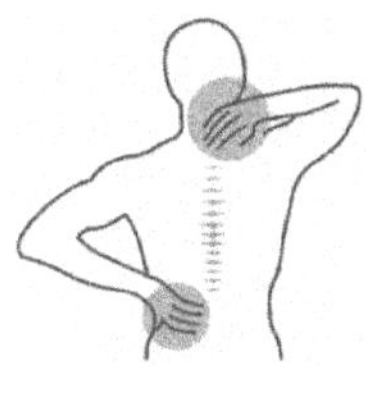

More About Shoes, Misinformation, and Society's Influence

- Not knowing what to do gives pain a license to rule. Reeducate yourself from the misinformation grip that makes you doubt your ability to break the cycles of chronic pain.
- Misinformation sets up low expectations. This means when you want to interrupt degeneration and pain, the wrong information says, "It's impossible; it can't be done."
- The body functions and changes by responding to the demands placed on it, from shoes, furniture, and exercise to how we breathe, sleep, eat, and think.
- No matter the length of time already spent in pain, you can find comfort and pain control by using your repair, recovery, and protective functions.

Step 8
Your Exercise Position

Set up your exercise position on the floor, couch, or bed. Use your exercise position to also nap, relax, read, watch TV, or visit with friends.

1. Support your body with a long upper body foam wedge to lie on. Use a head pillow to keep your chin from pointing to the ceiling, and use pillows under your arms to support arm weight.
2. Put your legs up on a chair with a king-size bed pillow on top, supporting your heels to the back of your thighs.
3. Slide a rolled towel or lumbar lengthener wedge just under your butt cheeks to angle the front of your hips toward your face to create an effortless pelvic tilt. The back of your waist should be resting on the wedge.

A little adjustment can make a big difference in pain relief. Feel the difference between supported heels and feet versus your feet hanging unsupported from the leg pillow.

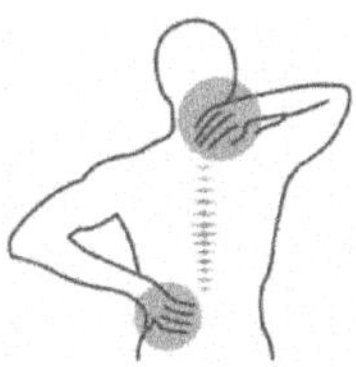

More About Your Exercise Position

- Supporting head weight takes ten to fifteen pounds of compressing pressure off your neck, shoulders, and spine.
- Sometimes using a hassock for lower leg height helps your hips if they are especially stiff.
- Remember that painful muscles have a hard time resting. Positioning supports take care of that for you.
- Supported exercise triggers pain relief responses and allows your muscles to work their rejuvenating magic.

Step 9
Pelvic Swing Breathing Exercise for Sexual Problems and Hip Pain

From a supported position, place your right hand on your right hip and your left hand on your left hip. Both elbows should be supported, and your eyes should be closed and covered.

1. Inhale and lift the back of your waist up into a comfortable arch position to shift the front of your hips down toward your feet. Hold the arch but not your breath until you need to let go and exhale.
2. Exhale to let the arch come back down to rest as the front of your hips tilt up toward your face.
3. After you exhale, breathe to catch your breath and let your lower breathing muscles (the muscles between your belly button and pubic bone on top of your belly) drop their weight into the cradle of your pelvis before inhaling again.

Pelvic swing breathing lifts the back of your waist from a resting position into the arch position to rotate your hips and exercise in a pain-free range of motion.

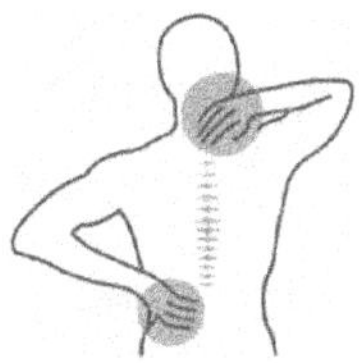

More About Pelvic Swing Breathing

- A supported pelvic tilt opens pathways for pain-free intercourse.
- Position yourself for pain-free penetration with a supported, effortless pelvic tilt.
- Supported exercise expands a pain-free range of hip socket motion.
- A supported pelvic tilt restores comfort at the pelvic floor region, which triggers a calming effect on your nervous system.

Step 10
Big Wave Breathing Exercise for Back Pain, Arthritis, and Depression

From a supported position of comfort, place one hand on your chest and the other lower down on your lower belly muscles between your belly button and pubic bone. Both elbows are supported; close and cover your eyes.

1. Inhaling to exercise the flexible length. Inhale for the expanding big wave muscle movement underneath your hands, picking up and lifting the bones of your ribs and spine. Hold the big wave expanded position, but not your breath. Breathe in and out, holding the expanded position.
2. See how long you can continue inhaling to expand your muscles so they lift and pull the bones they attach to and move.
3. Keep inhaling until you have to let go to exhale, and then breathe to catch your breath before beginning another long inhale.

The long inhale exercises muscle flexibility without stress or strain. Muscles that are fully expanded create room for the motions of rest, repair, and relaxation.

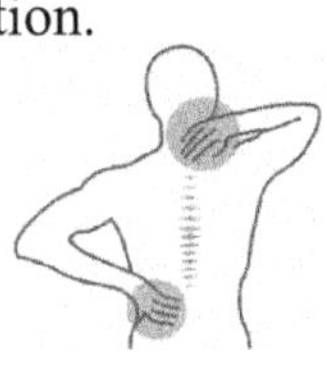

More About Big Wave Breathing Exercise

- Remember not to inhale into pain. Stay inside your comfort zone.
- With body weight supported, your diaphragm drops down and gives your lungs additional room to expand.
- Muscular breathing exercises your elastic lung capacity.
- By moving breathing muscles, your chest wall expands and delivers the motions that strengthen your body's vital capacity for life-force energy.
- The big wave breathing exercise releases the muscle tightness and restricted motion of back pain and allows lower back muscles to open and rest.
- Arthritis pain and inflammation are eased by the repeated, supported motions of the expansion of big wave breathing.
- Increased circulation brings oxygen into the bloodstream and helps lift depression.

Step 11
Placement Breathing Exercise for Discs, Sciatica, and Immune Enhancement

From a supported position of comfort, put both hands on your lower breathing muscles with fingertips toward each other and elbows supported on arm pillows. Close and cover your eyes.

1. With your tongue behind your top teeth, exhale a hissing sound and slowly pull down your lower breathing muscles underneath your hands into the cradle of your pelvis and close to your spine. Continue hissing out to press your lower back into the long foam body wedge your spine lies on to give your pelvis the freedom of movement to tilt up toward your face.
2. Hiss out until you can no longer hold that position, then let go and breathe to catch your breath.

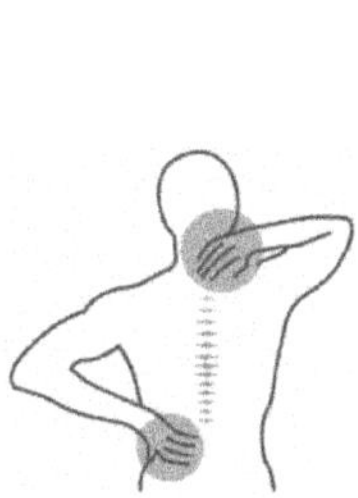

More About Placement Breathing

- As muscles move closer to bone, they squeeze the walls of lymph-carrying vessels to send lymph fluid to every cell in the body, thus boosting the immune system.
- Breathing muscles pull on vertebrae above and below the discs, providing the motion that delivers food and nutrition.
- Hissing acts as passive traction to lengthen and protect spinal bones from being too close to one another, which wears away disc fullness.
- Placement breathing returns space between the vertebrae up and down your spine. This matters because the sciatic nerve, made up of a bundle of fibers, needs room to exit your spine without the pain of being pinched.
- Exhale to place the back of your waist down toward the floor, which, in doing so, allows for an effortless pelvic tilt.

Step 12

Resting Breathing Exercise for High Blood Pressure and Fibromyalgia

Lie in a supported position of comfort with both hands resting on your body, elbows supported resting on pillows, and practice the following three breathing exercises.

1. How long can you inhale? Inhale, inhale, and inhale until you have to let go to exhale.
2. Exhale, and then breathe in and out, fast or slow, with your nose or mouth to catch your breath for easy, lazy breathing.
3. Breathe out easily for as long as possible after catching your breath until you have to inhale again.

Resting breathing gives thousands of breathing muscle fibers time to drop down into the cradle of your pelvis to rest close to your spine to spread, soften, rest, hang, open, repair, and recoup.

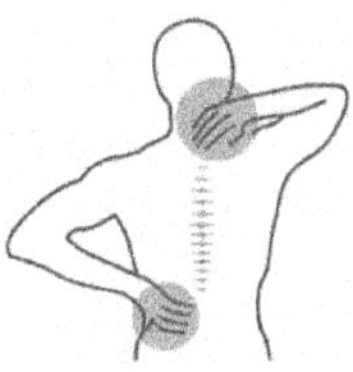

More About Resting Breathing Exercise

Resting breathing is the activity of muscular relaxation to bring your nervous system back to balance to calm stress.

- Resting breathing is physical rest, so connecting tissue reflexes can relax, which helps interrupt the restrictions of fibromyalgia.
- Resting breathing is relaxation training for all systems and functions of the body.
- Resting breathing is a healing response that exercises your body's ability to trigger itself for rest and repair. This allows the muscular walls of the arteries to better move and circulate blood, which lessens the burden on the heart muscle, aiding and reducing blood pressure.

Step 13

Arm Weight Circles for Scoliosis, Heart Problems, and Headaches

From a fully supported position of comfort, place the backs of both hands on top of each other and place them on your forehead. Cross one foot over the other and slide your legs closer to your body. Close and cover your eyes.

1. Place both hands on top of each other with your knuckles on your forehead. Slide your hands apart across your forehead until the back of your upper arms and elbows rest on the wedge. Take a long inhale.
2. Exhale and let your elbows and arms open out wide before circling down to cross your hands at your wrists to bring them up to rest your knuckles back on your forehead. Breathe to catch your breath.
3. Repeat #1 and #2.

Arm weight circles open the connecting tissue attachments of your ribs at your spine and sternum, expanding your chest wall for increased range of pain-free motion.

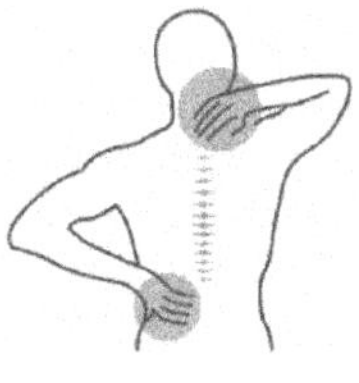

More About Arm Weight Circles

- Arm weight circles use the weight of your arms to open the many joints of your shoulder girdle to create space and room for the heart muscle and to relieve the constraints of scoliosis.
- Working the arms increases the pace of blood circulation to your heart muscle.
- Headaches are often traced to tight muscle attachments at the shoulder blades that remain in place too long.
- Constriction is a breeding ground for the buildup of pain.
- Arm weight circles provide the movements to clear waste products from muscle fibers, making the muscles more able to do their job.
- Scoliosis benefits from arm weight circles with a position support such as a tennis ball or paperback book under the hump to allow overstretched muscle fibers to settle closer to the bone.

Step 14

Leg-Shakes Exercise for Hamstring Injury, Neuropathy, and Varicose Veins

From a comfortable, supported position, slide one knee toward your chest. Keep your foot and calf on the leg pillow with your hand against your thigh closest to your chest.

1. Lift your heel up the thickness of one piece of paper, still touching the pillow. Hold that position until your leg muscles begin feeling the effort of supporting the weight of your leg.
2. Lift your heel an additional thickness of a piece of paper. Hold the new uplifted position. Hold, lift more, and continue to hold until you need to put your foot and calf down to rest on the pillow.
3. When your heel is lifted, let the shakes come if they do. Your knee should be bent, your foot and toes hanging softly. Repeat with the other leg.

Leg shakes transfer supported leg weight to leg muscle fibers for motions that access flexibility, build strength, and relieve pain.

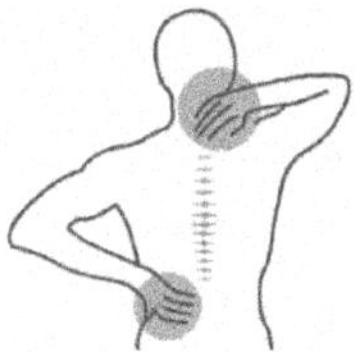

More About Leg-Shake Exercise

- Leg shakes soften hamstring tightness that restricts full, pain-free movement.
- Leg shakes improve the ability of the 26-foot bones and three ankle bones to provide better balance and stability.
- Legs are sometimes referred to as your second heart, because leg muscles pump blood through your veins and back to your heart and lungs for a fresh supply of oxygen.
- One job of the 13 long leg muscles is to push blood back up your legs against gravity, preventing the breakdown of veins and capillaries known as varicose veins.
- The motion of leg-shake exercises stimulates and feeds the nerve endings affected by neuropathy.

Step 15
Standing and Jiggling for Circulation, Leg Cramps, and Tension Release

Stand barefoot with feet parallel. Position each leg under the thigh bone attachment to the pelvis, which is less wide than your hips. Keep your toes, the outside of your feet, and your heels in solid contact with the floor.

1. Slightly bend both knees and press the bottoms of your feet into the floor, and jiggle up and down with your arches off the floor. Keep heels down on the floor. Knees stay soft as you jiggle up and down for a few minutes.
2. Continue jiggling and let your head and arms hang to the right, keeping the bottom of your feet in good contact with the floor. After a minute, jiggle back to center.
3. Let your head and arm hang to the left, keeping the bottom of your feet in good contact with the floor. After a minute, jiggle back to center.

Shaking motions help fear and trauma exit your tissues without leaving behind the scars of tightness and restricted motion. Trembling restores softness.

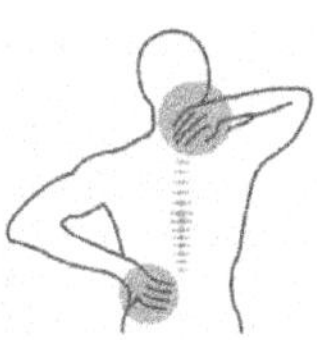

More About Standing and Jiggling

- If you press your feet harder into the floor, you can increase the jiggle intensity.
- Jiggling interrupts loss of movement from sustained muscle tension.
- The bounce of your jiggle increases the rate of both blood and lymph circulation.
- Cramps, pain, and fatigue inhibit the muscle's ability to meet required oxygen demands and clear waste products.

You’ve finished. Before you go …

Post/share that you finished this book.

Please star rate this book.

Reviews are solid gold to writers. Please take a few minutes to give us some itty bitty feedback.

ABOUT THE AUTHOR

Meg Margolis is a teaching instructor at Maggie Letvin's self-designed fitness program at Massachusetts Institute of Technology (MIT) in Cambridge, MA. Letvin's teaching style of anatomy, kinesiology, physiology, and human movement encouraged Meg to see beyond Maggie's incredible work, inspiring her to develop original exercises, including a positioning system for pain relief and physical repair that is now part of the fitness curriculum.

Harvard Medical School was Meg's first institutional client. Since 1976, she has taught community organizations, corporate groups, and individual clients in California. Her clients are referred by doctors, hospitals, and spine centers.

Meg has taught more than 2,000 patients how to move outside the confines of pain to recover physical ability with original exercises and a unique positioning system.

A partial list of California clients includes St. Mary's Spine Center, risk management programs for Marin County, Kaiser Permanente, the state of California, and Kaiser Workman's Compensation Fund.

To find out more about Meg Margolis and
Pain Relief Exercise, go to:
https://painreliefexercise.com

If you enjoyed this Itty Bitty™ book, you might also like…

- **Your Amazing Itty Bitty™ Guide to Cannabis** - Hyla Cass, M.D. and Mikayla Kemp

- **Your Amazing Itty Bitty™ Stress Reduction Book -** Denise Thomson, CHC

- **Your Amazing Itty Bitty™ Be the Boss Now** - Gregory Allan Datu Cendana

Or any of the many Amazing Itty Bitty™ books available online at www.ittybittypublishing.com

www.ingramcontent.com/pod-product-compliance
Lightning Source LLC
Chambersburg PA
CBHW072244240926
51846CB00012B/613
9781959964766